I0449950

THE ONLY PRESCRIPTION FOR HEALTHCARE REFORM

A Physician's Inside Perspective of the Real Problems Plaguing the System

Louis LoBalsamo M.D.

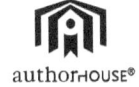

authorHOUSE®

AuthorHouse™
1663 Liberty Drive
Bloomington, IN 47403
www.authorhouse.com
Phone: 1-800-839-8640

© 2009 Louis LoBalsamo M.D. All rights reserved.

*No part of this book may be reproduced, stored in
a retrieval system, or transmitted by any means
without the written permission of the author.*

First published by AuthorHouse 9/1/2009

ISBN: 978-1-4490-2441-3 (e)
ISBN: 978-1-4490-2440-6 (sc)

*Printed in the United States of America
Bloomington, Indiana*

This book is printed on acid-free paper.

THE ONLY PRESCRIPTION FOR HEALTHCARE REFORM

A Physician's Inside Perspective of the Real Problems Plaguing the System

Louis LoBalsamo M.D.

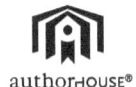

authorHOUSE®

AuthorHouse™
1663 Liberty Drive
Bloomington, IN 47403
www.authorhouse.com
Phone: 1-800-839-8640

© 2009 Louis LoBalsamo M.D. All rights reserved.

*No part of this book may be reproduced, stored in
a retrieval system, or transmitted by any means
without the written permission of the author.*

First published by AuthorHouse 9/1/2009

ISBN: 978-1-4490-2441-3 (e)
ISBN: 978-1-4490-2440-6 (sc)

Printed in the United States of America
Bloomington, Indiana

This book is printed on acid-free paper.

Dedicated to logic and
common sense; values I
hold dear to my heart.

Dedicated to my grandchildren
Amanda and Alyssa, and to all
my nieces and nephews; may our
leaders brighten their future.

A special dedication to my wife
Mary for her love and support.

COMMENT/WARNING

The Medical Profession is in shambles. Insurance Companies rule the market. Lawyers are gaming it for profit with no oversight. Most importantly, unless you are one of the lucky few left, whether you know it or not, your Primary Care is no longer being provided by a REAL Medical Doctor (M.D.). So wake up people and get the facts! Your livelihood is literally hanging in the balance.

CONTENTS

PREFACE

The state of the medical profession these days is in such disarray that unfortunately it appears that the demise of the real Primary Care Physician is inevitable. I say the "real physician" because society now appears to accept non-M.D.'s in the role of the Primary Care Provider.

Much of what I want to say will be somewhat autobiographical but is also intended to educate the reading public as to what an experienced M.D. from a humble background has to say about what they need to know during these troubled times. I have seen and experienced it first hand and it is now difficult for me to continue to sit back and not awaken this country to the reality of what they are experiencing everyday in the Medical Profession.

This unlengthy, yet concise narrative is meant to shed light to our leaders and the general public on the major issues crippling our healthcare delivery system here in the United States.

In my view, the problems aren't as complex and impalpable as everyone seems to think.

Therefore the analysis of the situation is quite simple and doesn't warrant a lengthy 500 page discussion. The solutions need some fine tuning but I will leave that to the people who were elected to do that job-the Congress and the President of the United States. I will propose some general ideas for solutions to the problems but that is not my goal here. My goal is to highlight the major problems. The solutions come easy once the real problems are known.

This document has no bibliography or footnotes. It references nothing but my personal opinions. These opinions are a result of my direct observations as a Physician within the Medical Profession itself. Obviously, I feel these are truths. The reader can decide the ultimate degree of credibility of my views.

1) With all due respect to the Law Profession and to all lawyers, it's time for you to reform your ways as well.

2) To all my Surgical and Procedural colleagues, as well as Insurance providers, it's time to recognize and reward the true value of Primary Care.

3) To the general public, it's time to become educated, engaged, and figure out what you truly desire.

4) To all my mid-level provider colleagues and friends, you are needed but your place I'm sorry to say is not at the forefront of Primary Care services.

INTRODUCTION

I am not a Democrat or a Republican. I am just a Physician who has plenty of experience seeing how the current broken medical care delivery system is practiced. I am an analytical person who sees the lack of logic pervasive throughout the system. During my well accomplished years working as a Primary Care Physician, I have directly viewed how my colleagues perform. I have seen the evolved standard of "defensive medicine" (I will define soon) that is ubiquitous within the system. The practice of defensive medicine is by far the costliest component jeopardizing our healthcare system. It has become so standard that even though the term is tossed around, it has become the hidden undercurrent threatening to overturn the boat and wash away the whole system. This standard is blindly accepted by society as the norm now. Our leaders ignore it. This defensive medicine that is grossly practiced is not one of the causes of the broken system, but rather a result of core issues that are wrong and need to be corrected.

"Defensive Medicine" needs to be defined now because the term will pop up diffusely (already has) throughout my discussion. What is defensive medicine? Essentially, defensive medicine is when a physician (after evaluation of a patient) orders a slew of very costly lab tests, radiology tests, procedures, and Consultants just because of the very slim chance that something uncommon or rare is going to be missed. The reality of the situation is that good physicians know that 99.9% of these tests and procedures will come back normal or confirm their initial clinical suspicion anyway. They order them anyway. Why? It's simple. They are afraid that they will get sued by patients and lawyers if they happen to miss the .1% chance of the wrong diagnosis. Why is this acceptable and why has the consumer and society in general let it become the standard of care? Does your plumber or car mechanic get it right more than 99.9% of the time? I understand we are dealing with people's lives here! Nevertheless, this standard is ridiculous. A good physician will concentrate most of his or her effort on getting a good medical history from the patient and performing a good comprehensive exam on the patient. In my experience, I have already been able to make the correct diagnosis at this point. If needed, only the minimal tests that may actually help you make or break a clinically suspected diagnosis should then be ordered. This is what I learned in Medical School and Internal Medicine Residency. This should be the accepted standard of care. If it was, there would be no fear of uncaged lawyers coming after you. Consequently, defensive medicine wouldn't exist. In fact, the standard I outlined and we have gotten away from should be promoted by society and accepted by the consumer. I am not saying that there are no legitimate malpractice, disability, or personal injury cases that deserve attention. Of course there are! However, there is a great deal of misleading fraud being practiced. Lawyers need to be caged and held accountable so that Physicians can get away from this ridiculous, out of control, and inflationary practice of defensive medicine. Society in general and the patient in particular, if they want affordable healthcare insurance that provides them access to high quality Primary Care Physicians, need to realize what currently is driving up insurance premiums and they need to begin to take responsibility and think twice before calling lawyers. The general public needs to be educated about what the reality is. Consumers of healthcare need to be part of our national healthcare reform. Patients need to be engaged in the solutions and determine what standard they want. We (everyone) cannot have it both ways. We either let good physicians do their job without fear of being sued, accept the standard that perhaps .1% of the time something may not be initially diagnosed correctly (even by the greatest physician), keep our premiums down, and prevent worsening of our healthcare crisis, or we continue the status quo, continue to promote the practice of defensive medicine, and let the healthcare delivery system chaos continue.

THE COMING EXTINCTION OF THE PRIMARY CARE MEDICAL DOCTOR (M.D.)

Unless the Primary Care Physician is properly placed at the top of the hierarchy of today's health care delivery puzzle, reimbursed accordingly, and recognized as the most important component to preventative health maintenance (which drives down health care costs in the long term), there is no incentive for myself or any other Primary Care Physician to enter practice again.

Enrollment into Internal Medicine/Family Medicine/Primary Care Residencies by medical school graduates is steadily declining. There is no incentive anymore for Primary Care. This society seems to think that Nurse Practitioners (3 years of superficial training) can deliver the same quality of care that good Board-Certified Internal Medicine doctors (7 years of intensive training) (like myself) can.

The insurance companies reimburse Primary Care services with peanuts compared to specialists. Who is the person more likely to contain costs by practicing preventative health maintenance-the surgeon (glorified technicians) or the Primary Care physician? This country has it all backwards. Why should I (in the role of a Primary Care physician) take the extra 1/2 hour needed to speak/educate/engage/ and promote well-being with the complicated or non-compliant diabetic patient (for example) if seeing 8 patients an hour and ignoring the health maintenance aspect (and the time needed to do so) gets me more reimbursement from the insurance companies? Why does this country think and insurance companies reimburse more for a ten minute cataract surgery than a 45 minute comprehensive, engaging, and educational experience the Primary Care physician can deliver? This is the essence of the problem! Surgeons get paid the most. They perform procedures but supply no prevention, are used primarily after diagnoses are made (rather than making diagnoses), and provide no quality treatment of chronic conditions. Obviously, surgeons have gone through rigorous training, but often end up serving as specialized technicians once medically trained personnel have already made the diagnosis. If you want to reform the system to contain costs in the long term by promoting good health maintenance and thereby avoiding disease, you must put into action a plan that gives incentives to and rewards the Primary Care physician the most! Emphasis should be on and the greatest reimbursement should be given to the Primary Care physician.

What is the difference between a Nurse Practitioner (N.P.) and a Medical Doctor (M.D.)? An N.P. is usually a nurse (R.N.) who goes for 2-3 years of additional training getting a little exposure to all the various common presenting medical problems or diagnoses, Yes, many patients present with "routine" problems that could indeed be handled satisfactorily by the N.P. But for every "routine" patient, there is one who presents the same way clinically but is far from "routine" and has other underlying complex diagnoses that need to be recognized and treated. These are the patients I believe the N.P. is not properly trained to handle. Diagnoses are missed and the patients suffer in the long run. Why then is society accepting the N.P. as becoming the standard for delivery of Primary Care? Every sector but the general public (the consumers themselves) knows why. The consumer or patient is just another pawn being used and many don't even know that they aren't seeing a REAL doctor. A Nurse Practitioner or a Physician Assistant is cheaper than paying a Physician. Insurance companies are reimbursing Primary Care already at ridiculously low rates. If I owned my own Primary Care practice/business, why then would I hire more M.D.'s?

The only reason that even Primary Care Practices have resorted to hiring mid-level providers (nurse practitioners, physician assistants) is purely financially based. Wouldn't everyone rather continue to see Board-Certified Primary Care Physicians? I bet our President does. With such de-emphasis on physicians (especially Primary Care Physicians) and poor respect and reimbursement by insurance companies for Primary Care services; of course mid-level providers (less costly) are being hired more and more at an alarming rate. There is certainly a role for mid-level providers to play in our healthcare system, but it is not at the forefront of Primary Care services. Perhaps the most useful role a mid-level provider could provide would be to assist Specialists once diagnoses are made. I will outline in this manuscript the differences in training that a Board-Certified Primary Care

Physician goes through as compared to Nurse Practitioners or Physician Assistants. The rest should be self explanatory. I have personally lived the experience. If this trend continues, more and more Primary Care Physicians (like myself) will opt out of office-based Primary Care and the Primary Care Physician will become extinct!

WHAT IT TAKES TO BECOME A BOARD-CERTIFIED PHYSICIAN

It now becomes important for the reader to understand what a person goes through after they have already graduated College to become a Physician is in stark contrast to what a Nurse Practitioner or Physician Assistant's education currently is. I am not here to denigrate my fellow Nurse Practitioner's or Physician Assistant's. But please do not pretend that the training of these professions is anywhere close to that of a Board-Certified Medical Doctor. This point directly emphasizes one of the core aspects of this book. Most of the public is not even aware of this.

Before I move on, I must explain to the general public what the training of an M.D. really entails. Let us go into the trenches now; at the front lines if you will. Then contrast this with the training of a Nurse Practitioner or a Physician Assistant. Now there are some

"Doctors" licensed to practice Medicine but they have not fulfilled the standard that is generally accepted amongst fully trained Board-Certified Physicians. Don't ask me how, but for some reason, the infinite wisdom of the State of New York allows a person trained in the United States who has completed Medical School but only one year of Residency (called Internship) to take a State exam and be licensed to practice Medicine. A foreign medical doctor or a foreign person with a Master's Degree in Biology can come into this country, not complete a Residency program, take an exam, and get licensed to practice Medicine. These people have limitations however because they have not completed an Accredited Residency Program. They are therefore not eligible for Board-Certification which is the highest achievement one can get in their field of medicine.

Now, let me not get to far ahead here because my ultimate goal is to explain the grueling task and time it takes to become a United States trained Board-Certified Medical Doctor (M.D.). This used to be the standard of care. This used to be what the Public demanded. This should be what the Public deserves.

Prior to the 1980's, the idea of the HMO (Health Maintenance Organization) did not exist. The business of Medicine was as usual. I entered Medical School in 1984, in debt of about $100,000 in loans already. So I picked an Accredited State University Medical School because it was relatively cheap. Who wanted another $150,000 in debt? I certainly didn't. My family didn't have the money. I was on my own financially. Remember, these were the costs back in the 1980's. Imagine what they are now! Medical School back then consisted of the first two years studying and learning various topics such as Anatomy or Physiology, and then taking tests. No courses in the Business of Medicine or the changing Evolution of Medicine. These tests were quite frankly boring and a bit tedious for me because it was all about memorizing a wealth of knowledge. But I managed. However, where was the Problem-Solving or intellectual challenge in this? Nevertheless, this was not an easy task. The lack of any training in the Business side of Medicine or even the knowledge that things were changing in the outside world put all of us in an isolated bubble that we wouldn't escape until going into Practice. The third and fourth years of Medical School finally involved clinical training with actual patients. This was both good and bad. Obviously, the whole point was to actually learn how to care for patients. What the general public doesn't understand is what this training actually consisted of. During clinical rotations, you would be part of a team, moving up the ladder as expected, taking on more responsibility as you go along, and taking on a workload that defies human nature. Your life would basically be consumed for those two years and you hadn't even started Residency or even become an M.D. yet. It was during these two years that I thought Internal Medicine and ultimately a self-owned private Practice in Primary Care Medicine was the course for me. Where else could I use my common sense and "Problem-Solving" capabilities to its fullest potential? I took a year leave to do medical research to find something intellectually challenging, published a few papers in conjunction with another Physician, and then went back to finish my clinical duties. Finally I graduated and obtained my Medical Degree. But wait. It hadn't even started yet. So far, four years of College and four years of Medical School and I wasn't even done yet. Wait until you hear what Residency training was like. Meanwhile, the Business of Medicine and the strangle-hold of "third parties" are evolving in the outside real world but I am too involved in my training to stay ahead of the curve.

The next step is to apply and get into an Accredited Residency Program in Internal Medicine. I did and was accepted. I actually stayed in the Consortium where I trained during Medical School. It was familiar. You make out of something what you put into it. Why move anywhere else? Looking back, I wish I would have at least left New York State where HMO's, Lawyers, and Insurance Companies were making their stand quickly and decisively.

First year of Residency is called Internship. A full 3 years is required to fulfill an Internal Medicine Residency. Once someone completes the three years and all its requirements, only then is that person eligible to achieve the highest distinction in Internal Medicine which is "Board-Certification". The preparation of this exam itself takes about one year to do it right. Then you take the American Board of Internal Medicine exam and hope for the best (i.e. pass the exam). What I have just outlined is a simple summary of four years of your life invested even after you have achieved the M.D. degree. Now let's take a step back and describe some of the details one must go through during these four years.

Internship begins in July and ends in June. As the first year Resident, you are given the largest more direct patient care load. It is your duty to screen all the patient situations and then present them to your Senior Resident for a treatment plan. Once the treatment plan is in place, it is your job to take care of all the little details which include writing the history and physicals, tracking down all the lab results, doing all the procedures no one else wants to do, drawing blood if others can't, tracking down family members, and getting the case ready to present in an acceptable manner to your Attending Physician (the person in the superior position to the Senior Resident and ultimately responsible for all patient care) the following morning. A typical schedule for an Intern and in fact the whole Residency team (at least when I was training) would be 36 hours of continuous care during which you are admitting to the hospital upwards to 20 patients overnight, following all the other patients assigned to your team who are in the hospital already admitted, and writing daily notes on all these patients. Then you would have to present all the newly admitted overnight cases to your Attending with the whole team present in the morning usually. When you are done after the 36 hours, you get to go home, eat, sleep, show up the following morning and repeat the whole 36 hour process all over again. This goes on for a whole year! Looking back, it is amazing how anyone can function during this time. I must admit however, that the first year of my Residency or during this "Internship", I probably learned the greatest percentage of patient care that I still retain today. However, there are so many negatives that this process condones. Some of these include ignoring your own health (since you have no time to think of yourself). Examples of this include learning poor behavior patterns when it comes to eating, sleeping, exercising, and taking time for spiritual growth. By the way, your personal growth and well-being outside your own medical team is in reality of no interest to anyone in the system. As you move up the "food-chain" (second and third years), you slowly take on more of a teaching and supervisory role within the team. But the hours are the same, the system doesn't change, and the behaviors of ignoring oneself become more entrenched within you. The irony of a physician spending all your time caring for others while ignoring your own health is perplexing and the

Medical Establishment is definitely an enabler in this process. What hypocrisy! Without realizing how many years have passed, what you have evolved into, and how much the world has changed, you finally finish Residency. You then take and hopefully pass the Board Exam, and you are now ready to break out of the "bubble" and enter the "real" world of Medicine.

Now contrast all of the above with the educational schedule to obtain a Nurse Practitioner license. After High School, one could go for 2 years of training for the usual R.N. (Registered Nurse) degree. The Nurse Practitioner portion involves 3 more years of superficial textbook and clinical exposure to all the various fields of Medicine. Then you are done after taking an exam to get your license. Society then allows you to flow right into a Primary Care role for about 60-80% of the average net salary of a Board-Certified Internal Medicine Doctor. Somehow, even with the slight disparity in income, I find it hard to see the equivalence between the training programs that ultimately lead to the M.D. versus the N.P. degree. Some N.P.'s would argue that there is more to the picture such as the requirement (at least currently in New York State) of a Physician reviewer of their care. All this means is that the

State requires the physician to periodically audit patient charts of the Nurse Practitioner and sign off on them. The physician doesn't even have to be physically present during the care of a patient provided by the N.P. As I write this, there is a growing movement amongst Nurse Practitioners and their lobbyists for complete autonomy from the physician. Some want to start private practice groups of their own believing that they can provide the same or better Primary Care than the M.D. even without the M.D.'s oversight. I beg to differ. Simple common medical ailments and diagnoses will likely be treated similarly; but many underlying, complicated, or rare diagnoses will be missed. Patients won't know the difference and they will ultimately suffer. The money saved by the Insurance company by reimbursing a N.P. instead of an M.D. for one of these "atypical" patients will eventually be spent (if not more) later on down the line for illness that could have been avoided if a good properly trained M.D. had been involved from the start. Insurance companies, however, are short-sided and won't see this long-term issue coming. They will simply be concentrating on containing short-term costs. The net effect of all this will be increased (not decreased) medical expenditure, negative outcomes for patients, and certainly not reform for the better.

GREED, UNREGULATED LAWYERS, AND THE EVOLUTION OF "DEFENSIVE MEDICINE"

THE ROOT PROBLEM!

It is quite clear that the cost to provide medical care to people in this country has grown exponentially and has crippled our economic system. This is true even despite the fact that millions of people do not have medical insurance. This fact itself (people not having insurance) contributes enormously to the problem of out of control costs.

The real issue here is how this country got to this situation in the first place. I believe to unravel the problem itself, it is essential to understand the evolution of the problem. Many years ago when lawyers and insurance companies were not involved in the patient-physician relationship; when the profession of medicine was respected by the public and viewed as prestigious; the only concern the patient and the patient's family had was to be treated and hopefully get better. The only concern on the part of the physician was to sincerely do what he/ she felt was justifiably best to help the patient. Regardless of the outcome, the patient, the family, and the Physician were content with the attempt at the medical care given and the patient and family were appreciative most of the time. Then came along the insurance companies and the biggest culprit of all, the lawyers. Rightfully so, there was a market for medical insurance so this evolved but initially remained outside the patient-physician relationship. Physicians determined what was necessary and these services were billed. Insurance companies would simply reimburse for services like any other insurance industry. Insurance for people's families was affordable and provided through employees as a work benefit at a time when any type of work was seen as necessary and people worked with a sense of pride because they were providing for their families. Why was insurance easily provided by employees and affordable for workers at this time? Because no third parties were instigating the patient-physician relationship. Therefore, the need to play "defensive medicine" by Physicians did not exist. By my estimate, in today's world, "defensive medicine" unfortunately now defines the profession. I will proceed further in defining "defensive medicine" and why it evolved soon but this will become quite clear as this brings us to our next most important point.

Most people in this country want the freedoms the constitution provides and minimal government intrusion into their life. Obviously, government is unquestionably needed for such basic things as military protection, establishment on a large scale of models for supplying basic needs as education, police protection, etc. Whether or not government should be involved in other things not so undeniable is the question. We all want Capitalism to work. It cannot work however without some sort of regulation. Should the government provide this regulation? Well, who else will? To understand some of the problems we face now, one must understand the innate behavioral instincts of man; human behavior if you will. At the core of this are such simple characteristics or instincts of mankind that have evolved. One of these is greed. Plain and simple, if gone unchecked, in general, man's natural progression is to let the greed surface. I'm not saying that everyone is greedy. There are many in this world that do selfless things to help others. Let's face it though; man's natural tendency is to be greedy. This is why regulatory systems or programs are needed and ideally should be provided by people elected to represent them. In this country, that would be the legislative and executive branches of the government. Our government is far from perfect. We however at least have the option to vote people out that we feel are not selfless and do not represent us. Why have we seen an economic collapse recently in our country? The answer at the heart of this is greed. How was this greed able to surface? The answer to this is lack of regulation. The same holds true with our healthcare system. In fact, it is quite analogous to what happened with the economy. The healthcare crisis however has been going on for a much longer period of time.

Now I know what I'm about to say may irritate lawyers in general (I know people who are lawyers and even our President is one) but the truth of the matter is that lawyers have been gaming the medical establishment for years. I am convinced through general observation of this. I am also convinced that the general public feels the same way in that some lawyers definitely influence this healthcare mess; they just don't know the details. The effect of lawyers being able to "game" the system is the root of the problem and the ultimate reason why healthcare costs have skyrocketed. Why have lawyers been able to do this? They are not regulated and being held accountable. They have flooded the airwaves and internet with commercials, established small loose local associations with insurance companies and judges, created their own system of deals where most lawsuits can be "settled" out of court, have become adept at misrepresentation of issues, have misled and perhaps provided illegal tactics, whereby everyone wins and gets a piece of the pie. The general idea is to set up a system so that it is not cost-effective for any persons or groups involved to see the lawsuit all the way through trial; unless it is one of the 10-20% (I'm estimating based on experience) of cases that are truly legitimate. The other 80-90% of the cases are nebulous at best and sometimes frivolous. The system however still allows for these 80-90% of cases to be "settled" out of court because it is more cost-effective and less time consuming for all involved. Even when a lawsuit without merit is brought against a physician, he or she is usually told just to settle out of court. Otherwise, it will be time consuming, not cost-effective, and may expose the physician's name and ultimately ruin that physician's reputation (even if he or she did absolutely nothing wrong and provided the standard of care accepted within the community). Physicians do what they are told. Who wants their reputation dragged through the mud (even when you are completely confident you did nothing wrong)? After all, isn't this why malpractice insurance exists? The analogy to the current economic crisis is clear. Lawyers are to the healthcare crisis as deregulation of Wall Street and Bankers are to the economic crisis.

While greed in all its forms is the fuel that drives the engine of all sectors of our healthcare system today, it is the unregulated business of law and specifically lawyers that is the ultimate evil in the process that got everything out of hand. Greed, of course, influences all components (including the patient or consumer) of our healthcare delivery system; not just lawyers. I will discuss this elsewhere. However, at some point, lawyers realized that there was a market (in society) to convince consumers of medical care that malpractice could be going on and therefore whenever there was a negative outcome, there was a justifiable reason to always investigate the physician's actions.

Probably the most important root cause problem driving up healthcare costs is the standard of practicing defensive medicine. With the lack of oversight, unaccountability, deceit, fraud, and general manipulation of the public and the Medical Profession that our current Law Profession is so pervasively doing, who can blame physicians for practicing defensive medicine? Physicians know that despite their great intentions and how well they do; they can be sued at any given moment regardless of the quality of care they provide. This directly has forced the evolution of defensive medicine.

Lawyers knew that in their unregulated, bureaucratic, and sometimes corrupt industry, they could make large amounts of money regardless of the quality and substance of the claim. This began the unraveling of the independent patient-physician relationship. It began the process of demeaning the medical profession. Society no longer looked at Physicians with hope and prestige. Now society had a vehicle to sue physicians. It became all about how the physician did some wrong. So naturally the response by the medical profession was to start ordering tests that weren't really needed, having patients follow up with them more frequently which isn't needed most of the time, sending patients to as many consultants as they could think of even though the Primary Care Physician already had the competence to deal with the patient's problem, and spending lots of time documenting and writing down notes instead of spending more time questioning and examining patients. There are other behaviors now that dominate the provision of medical care by Primary Care Physicians but what I have explained is essentially the definition of "defensive medicine" and how it evolved. One could look at it this way. When a Physician is doing things and ordering things with a main goal in mind to protect himself/herself from a lawsuit(by making it look to the layperson and the legal system that "everything" was done) instead of primarily focusing on the only TRUE needs of the patient, he/she is practicing "defensive medicine". This now dominates the culture to an unbelievable extent that only those of us "inside" the culture truly see it. Society, in its blindness, sees this as the normal way of doing things. Most patients have no clue that they are being sent to consultants or for testing that is really not needed (but they complain why their insurance premiums are going up). Patients also see their bills and actually think that the physician has determined the charges and the fee schedules for services. Patients are blind to the fact that these prices are defined by reimbursement schedules set by the insurance companies. Primary Care Physicians are especially vulnerable to insurance company policies and in fact get no where near the reimbursement that is charged on these bills. Do you think patients know this? It is quite clear they don't. It is very hard for a physician like myself to continue to operate in a climate like this. I have left Primary Care because of this. I agree there should be a standard of care that all physicians meet. But who defines this standard? I certainly don't believe that lawyers, the legal system, or insurance companies should be setting this standard. The only thing they have caused is a broken patient-physician relationship.

Insurance companies should be secondary and not primarily controlling the market or the patient-physician relationship. Lawyers need to be caged and also held accountable for all the frivolous lawsuits they bring driving up the price of health care. Fine them when they bring a malpractice lawsuit with no substance! They do this now because there is no oversight and they know the "system" will allow for a settlement (regardless of the substance of the lawsuit) because it is cheaper to "settle" than to bring all these lawsuits to court. We practice preemption from a national security standpoint with all our nuclear missiles around the world. Why not practice preemption regarding medical-liability issues with these lawyers? I bet you this would contain costs tremendously!

THE REACTIONARY RESPONSE BY THE MEDICAL INSURANCE INDUSTRY, THE BIRTH OF THE "HMO", AND WHAT PUBLIC OPTIONS NEED TO ADDRESS

This brings me to the next step in the evolution of the medical care industry. Once physicians began to collectively practice "defensive medicine" to ward off lawsuits, the costs of medical care skyrocketed. The natural response to this by the insurance companies who were now no longer making a large profit on all their policies was to interject themselves in the process and try to "manage the care". Without addressing the real problem of an out of control legal system driving up the costs by bringing substantial frivolous lawsuits, the birth of the HMO (Health Maintenance Organization) by the insurance industry occurred. Because of the historical employee-based provision of medical care, the insurance industry knew they had already cornered and controlled the marketplace providing medical insurance to families (since most people need to work to provide for their families) so they were now in the position to disrupt the patient-physician relationship and use their power to now attempt to dictate how medical care was going to be prescribed. This was their grand plan to attempt to drive down costs by pushing physicians to follow policies written by them. Unfortunately, everyone working at these insurance companies including the high level positions and all the people writing restrictive policies were a breed of business people with absolutely no background or clue as to what was medically appropriate and what was not medically appropriate. More so, they were just reacting and still are just reacting to what physicians are doing without realizing that what physicians are doing is just the evolutionary byproduct of the legal system (lawyers) interjecting and driving the motor of "defensive medicine". I never could understand why it was and still is so difficult for CEO's of insurance companies to see this. A better solution might be to concentrate on how lawyers are affecting the delivery of medical care and perhaps concentrate their efforts on this. Somehow though, things have evolved to the point where everyone wants to point their finger and efforts at the physician whom has now become the "bad guy/gal".

I do agree with the concept that everyone in this nation should have affordable medical insurance. I would go as far as saying that this should be mandated but only if the root causes of the system's failure are fixed. The current public options of Medicaid and Medicare do not work the way they are structured today. Therefore, just expanding this type of health care service to cover the uninsured is not the answer. The system needs a complete overhaul with an emphasis on Primary Care reimbursement and incentive to deliver wellness, prevention, and proper chronic disease management. This by itself, if third party interfering is rooted out, will evolve a system that inherently brings down costs of healthcare. There is currently no incentive for Primary Care Physicians to deliver care to patients that have insurance that reimburses the Physicians less than private insurance providers. Private insurance companies have a long way to go themselves to get it right. They feel they can somehow inject themselves into the doctor-patient relationship and "manage care". This does not work. There are too many loopholes and too much wasted money and resources. This is not their rightful place anyway. The private insurance companies are simply dealing with the bottom line which is making a profit. They pretend to be patient advocates but they are not. They are just businesses reacting to multiple forces they have no control over (similar to what physicians are dealing with). Again, without properly dealing with the root causes of our divided and fragmented healthcare system, cost cannot be contained. Insurance companies will just continue to remain reactionary and premiums will continue to go up.

Everyone needs medical insurance that provides for quality service. This quality service will only be delivered by Primary Care Physicians in the office setting if they are properly reimbursed for their time and efforts with an emphasis on wellness, prevention, and good chronic disease management. When people are uninsured or the system essentially blocks them from getting good quality Primary Care because they have undesirable insurance such as Medicaid or Medicare, they will continue to only use Emergency Rooms and walk-in-clinics when they become ill. This is a huge cost containment issue for the healthcare system. Any mandated public option insurance needs to reimburse Primary Care Physicians on an even keel with Private Insurers. Then you will get true competition and the spirit of Capitalism between all insurance companies including the public options.

Having a government run public option to get all uninsured people coverage is a good concept. However, it will not work if the underlying real issues aren't addressed. It will mimic Medicare for people under age 65. If reimbursement for real Primary Care Physicians is not increased and truly placed at the forefront of health care with its ability to prevent disease and manage chronic medical conditions with efficiency without the role of defensive medicine hanging over its head, it will not contain costs in the long run and will not look attractive for Primary Care Physicians. These patients will be treated like current Medicare patients are (put at the bottom of the list to enroll in your practice) because it will not be cost effective to take on this population. Of course the American Medical Association would be against this option if the above issues aren't addressed. They also have their own ideas and political agenda. Private insurers will always be against any publicly funded basic healthcare coverage they are scared they will not be able to compete and will lose business. Does anyone really think private HMO's want to see reform of the current system?

LEAVING PRIMARY
CARE MEDICINE

I am a twice Board-Certified (1997, 2007) Internal Medicine Physician with 17 years experience in the profession. My record and local reputation is impeccable. I have spent 15 of those 17 years practicing Primary Care Medicine. For reasons that will become apparent in this document, I left Primary Care and am now practicing full-time as a salaried Hospital Physician concentrating my efforts treating the acutely ill population. During my time in Primary Care, I have essentially split my years between the private sector and Veteran population (as a government employee). I have experienced almost all types of administrative bureaucracies whether it be within my profession or dealing with insurance companies. When I entered medical school here in the United States in 1984, "managed care" (or more commonly known as the "HMO") insurance did not exist (at least to any significant degree). When I finished my Internal

Medicine Residency here in the United States in 1992, the "HMO" (or Health Maintenance Organization) had exploded onto the scene and was quickly sequestering the health insurance market. This was being provided mainly as an employee-related benefit (as health insurance had traditionally been provided). As an effort to control costs, reimbursement for Primary Care Physicians was at this time (and still is) being reduced. Primary Care Physicians (especially the isolated ones) and hospitals (especially the smaller community hospitals) quickly scrambled to unite in an attempt to gain power to negotiate better contracts with the almighty HMO's. It became clear that my personal dream of opening a solo practice was no longer a viable option from a business perspective. Therefore, I initially joined a small group of private physicians that, though small in numbers on a national level, had a rather significant presence in the local community. After about 6 years in the private sector with managed care gaining strength, taking over the market, interfering more and more into the patient-physician relationship, lowering reimbursement, and making it intolerable to practice good medicine and paradoxically "health maintenance" (example: requiring you to see 6-8 patients an hour; some of them with multiple medical problems), I left the private sector and joined the local Veterans Administration Medical Center as a full-time practicing Primary Care Physician providing both outpatient and inpatient care to our Veteran Heroes. I worked at the Veteran's Hospital for nine years.

Despite their assumed good intentions but unfortunate lack of foresight, ultimately the misuse by Administration of the electronic database (i.e. the electronic medical record itself), the abuse and the inevitable negative effects of the electronic medical record system that the Veteran's Hospital adopted (which I will detail and explain soon along with its implications in the private sector) became standards I could no longer ethically observe or be part of. I therefore resigned and lost my desire to practice as a Primary Care Physician.

ELECTRONIC MEDICAL RECORDS

BE AWARE!

I worked at the local Veteran's Hospital for nine years providing Primary Care Medicine to our Veteran Heroes. This VAMC happens to have led the process (locally) of electronically converting the medical records of patients. When I began, everything was still on paper. When I resigned, almost everything was electronic within the regional Veteran's Hospitals. The records could only be accessed within the system and not by the Private Sector. I can pass on to you directly the effects and the evolutionary details of the pros and cons. I "lived" this and have first hand knowledge everyone needs to know. My concerns are that the "cons" are inevitable and in my opinion do not outweigh the benefits; especially if the evolving Government mandate of the use of electronic medical records (EMR's) is taken nationally via the Web. At my local VA, the "cons" and their indirect negative effect on the Patient-Physician relationship is what ultimately made me resign. Ironically, it was the fact that I cared too much about the patients that I had to leave them.

I could go on for a very long time with details but I'm going to get to the few main potential "cons" that worry me. Obviously, there are many "pros" to having an electronic record and everyone including the President's Advisors is pointing this out. There is a place for electronically converting records but I believe the line needs to LITERRALY be drawn at the door (of the Physician's office, of the Hospital, of the Insurance companies, etc.). Integrating these records over the Web will create problems that no one wants to concentrate on now because the emphasis is on cost containment right now. This is what happened at my local VA. I forecasted the problems that would arise but none of my administrators was willing to stop and re-evaluate the situation. They had a mandate from the previous Administration in Washington, D.C. and they were carrying out that mandate blindly like you would expect a true bureaucracy does. The problem is essentially that the issue wasn't FULLY thought out before implemented. I would encourage this country not to make the same mistake.

Once again, the intent of the program at the VAMC may have been to improve things. Nevertheless, even though the data may look good, the patient care suffered. Here are just a few of the serious adverse results of what happened at my local VA. When your electronic system goes down, you cannot proceed treating patients. When the emphasis is on keeping the electronic database and templates up to date for other purposes besides the M.D.'s own necessary needs for patient care (in a setting where you need to see 5-6 patients an hour), the physician spends the whole visit "treating the computer" and not the patient. This became the "running joke", if you will. Other providers openly would just come right out and say how they were "treating the computer". It was becoming a ridiculous, unethical, and poorly managed patient-care environment. This was the first step in my decision to leave. How do you treat patients without engaging them, speaking with them, educating them, taking a good history, performing a full focused exam, discussing results, speaking with family members, etc?

Some physicians weren't even getting up from their chair. They spent all the time "treating the computer" and guess what; they were the ones that looked like "good" providers because their patient databases were more up to date and this data was all the administrators cared about. This was so obviously the definition of bureaucracy. Leave it up to the Government to lead the way. The "last straw" for me that made me ultimately resign was when Administration decided to use this database (a database never created for any other purpose than to communicate medical history better) to determine "pay for performance" for physicians as part of their salary. Some physicians began to "catch on" and input false or "made-up" information into the computer record just to satisfy poorly determined outcome measures so that they would get their "pay for performance" in full. What a disgusting and immoral thing to do! Whether you realize it or not, this actually also affects patient care. Hypothetically speaking, as an example, if a Primary Care Physician falsely inputs into the record that a patient had a colonoscopy "in the private sector" within the last 5 years, another physician (example: an Oncologist working up anemia) looking at the record (during another appointment) will assume the colonoscopy was really done and may not inquire about it. I've seen it happen!

When the Federal Government/VA decided to pay me based on "performance measures", it began to paradoxically affect patient care by taking valuable time away from me and my patients (because I had to sit at the computer updating the patient databases). I was not about to compromise my ethics! I could have "gone with the flow" just so I would get my "performance pay", but that is not my nature. I tried to work it out with my Administrators but by that time, they just didn't want to hear it anymore. I was just too outspoken for them trying to do the RIGHT thing! I had to resign.

When an electronic record is used for the correct purposes and is 100% confidential, it is a great thing. What happened at my previous job at the VAMC will happen in the Private Sector. Insurance companies will begin reimbursing physicians based on an arbitrary "performance measure" database without READING THE RECORD and this will lead to paradoxical effects and poor medical care. What is worth more in a non-compliant uneducated diabetic patient for example? Should the physician get paid based on whether that patient's HgbA1C (a measure of diabetes control) is under a certain number (lower values are better) or should that physician get paid for the 1 hour of time spent speaking with the patient, explaining things to the patient, educating the patient, emphasizing the importance and implications of good diabetes control, etc? What will ultimately happen is that physicians will either refuse to see these types of patients (ones that take time to EDUCATE) or falsify data one way or the other (like what I observed with my own eyes at the VA). Also, with regards to confidentiality, we all know that the Internet is not 100% reliable and never will be. That is why electronic medicalrecords need to remain "at the door".

Our Federal Government is pushing for a national electronic medical record system with all its "perks". I have described above the negative outcomes that might occur. I have also learned recently from the news that questions are already surfacing as to how safe someone's records are on-line. Apparently, by just searching pharmacy and insurance company bills on the Internet, someone can access private medical information about you. At least it can be inferred based on the medications listed or the diagnostic codes listed.

Once again I must reiterate that an electronic medical record system can be very valuable and less costly in the long run but it must be used properly and must remain secure for only physicians to use.

Putting into place the accessibility of EMR's over the Internet will violate Federal Privacy Laws such as "HIPPA" (Health Information Protection and Portability Act). Workers on all levels in physician's offices, hospitals, nursing homes, or insurance companies will be able to obtain private medical data on anyone under the "guise" of medical necessity. There is no way this will be able to be monitored 100% on a National level. We have already seen security infringements and stolen data on a much lower scale within the VA system; even though they continue to strive for complete privacy.

True intelligence is being able to recognize the potential negative outcomes of a mandate and weigh them against the positive aspects before that mandate is implemented. The short term positive benefits are easy to see. It takes intelligence and foresight to see the future negative outcomes that will occur.

GREED AND THE
OTHER PLAYERS

Let us go back to the problem of greed and discuss how it affects each component of our healthcare system today before we discuss possible simple, yet definitive solutions to the problems we face today.

The innate and unfortunate human personality trait of greed in a market without oversight and regulation, within our Capitalistic society, is a recipe for abuse, danger, and disaster. I am not a Communist. However, pure unregulated Capitalism does not work. A clear example of this is our current economic crisis. There must be some independent oversight to make sure people are "playing by the rules". Whether government or a private sector regulatory body does this doesn't matter. The point is that it must be done and whatever model is most independent, efficient, and uncorrupt should be utilized.

How does greed currently play out in all sectors of our healthcare system? I have already discussed at length the effect of the unregulated law profession so I won't reiterate that here. Let's move on to the consumers or the patients. Knowing there are hundreds of lawyers on the sidelines advertising and waiting to sue doctors, hospitals, and pharmaceutical companies, in conjunction with all the information available to them on the Internet (some of which is false or inaccurate), family and friends telling them what tests they "heard" the patients should have, lack of education by their physician (remember, the Primary Care Physician has no time to do this under the current reimbursement system), lack of self-education (real education), the consumer presents himself or herself to the doctor demanding antibiotics, drugs, or tests (many times not indicated). The consumer has paid their high insurance premium and feels entitled to get whatever he or she wants; without any regard to the system as a whole. This is how the patient or consumer currently displays their greed.

Let's now discuss the insurance companies and how their greed plays out. Well, this is quite simple. As I have mentioned elsewhere, they are just private businesses trying to make a profit. There is nothing wrong with this. What is wrong is at what point is this profit unreasonable and detrimental to society and its citizens? At what point are they abusing the consumer; raising premiums so that CEO's can make millions? Remember, they pretend to be patient advocates but have really devoted personnel behind the scenes to simply figure out how to contain costs and spend less on behalf of the consumer.

What about the Pharmaceutical Industry? This industry is simply out of control. They spend so much money on lobbyists to influence politicians and the Federal Drug Administration (FDA) to push their new drugs to market so quickly (as if we need more drugs in this country) with some being recalled in a year. The recalls don't matter to them because that is already figured in to the cost effectiveness of their marketing program. I am not against researching and developing new, better, and less toxic medications that are much needed to treat specific medical conditions that do not currently have adequate and safe treatment. However, how many drugs (within the same class of drugs) do we really need to treat common problems such as hypertension, heart disease, diabetes, emphysema, arthritis, (I could go on)? As a physician, I know that I can personally manage these conditions with probably about one-quarter of the current drugs available. Instead of continuing to manufacture different versions of drugs that are already available, why doesn't the pharmaceutical industry spend more of its resources developing medications that actually cure problems? The answer is obvious. They have no interest in curing disease. This would just eventually put them out of business.

Now what about physicians? Are they perfect? Absolutely not. Are some of them greedy? Of course some are. The question I propose though is how much of this greed (where there truly is greed) is purposeful or secondary and reactionary to all of the other greedy forces exerting pressure on doctors? Also, I do believe that most physicians are good people, not greedy, care about patients, morally just, and simply trying their best. There is an overwhelming myth in this country that all physicians are millionaires (or very rich). Maybe some Specialists are. I have been a Primary Care Physician for fifteen of my seventeen years in the profession and I can honestly tell you that I am certainly not a millionaire. I must say it again! Primary Care Physicians are being busted out of the system as it stands and works today. Let's get rid of the consciously immoral and greedy physicians but let's recognize that most are good people and just fighting the system to stay afloat; especially the good quality and fully credentialed Primary Care Physician.

GET RID OF
DEFENSIVE MEDICINE!

So how do we get ourselves out of this mess? For me, the answers are simple and logical. As previously mentioned, I'm not going to dwell on the details. Some may feel that what I will generally propose is naïve and cannot occur at this point in our complicated society. I challenge them (and all of us) to start by looking in the mirror and recognize the greed in their lives. Acknowledge your own personal greed and the greed all around you. Then do something about it and stop living this life so selfishly. Once we face our greed, we can start unraveling the layers of complexity in the healthcare system that have evolved over the years.

The solutions become clear once we understand the problems that evolved to cause this healthcare mess. Instead of adding many new layers of complexity in an attempt to fix the system, why not just address the problems that got us here? I do believe that some spending by the Federal Government is needed. However, if we peel off the problematic layers that already exist, this will result in an unparalleled degree of cost-containment that will undoubtedly exceed the level of government spending needed. This is the true bipartisan approach. The net effect will be to reverse and reduce the levels of healthcare spending that exist today and give everyone in this country the ability to obtain affordable healthcare coverage.

Defensive Medicine must end! Therefore, we must devise a plan to educate the public and most importantly regulate the Law Profession. Yes, everyone in this country should have the freedom to pursue an injustice if they have experienced one. On the other hand, if the system allows anyone to hire a lawyer and pursue a claim without true merit, the chaos will continue. So where do we draw the line? I believe that if the general public understands how the current practice of defensive medicine (driven by the fear of litigation) is driving up their insurance premiums, some people may think twice about approaching lawyers with lawsuits that may not have real substance. I understand that the general public is not uniformly versed in malpractice law. This doesn't mean they can't be educated about the current system and engaged in ways to reform it.

This is why we need to primarily regulate the Law Profession. After all, as previously discussed, members within the Law Profession currently are the root of all evil.

Over the years, lawyers identified the market, manipulated it, and are progressively gaming it for their own greedy purposes. All of this continues without oversight. We must put in place incentives for lawyers to "think twice" as well.

For the sake of example, let's split up malpractice, disability, and personal injury claims or lawsuits into three categories. The first category would be claims that are frivolous or without sufficient merit. The second category would be borderline cases. The third category would be claims with definite substance. Now add regulatory features such as possible fines or penalties on lawyers for proceeding with frivolous lawsuits. This would certainly put them on notice that manipulating and gaming the system with empty claims will not be tolerated and will negatively affect them. Now the lawyers must think twice. With the probability of facing a fine or penalty, lawyers will not pursue anymore the first category of claims described above. All of a sudden, the burden on our healthcare system of a large number of claims goes away. What a cost-reducing measure this would be!

For the second category of claims, one possible answer could be to create local Arbitration Councils composed of independent, respected, and law-abiding citizens representing different sectors of society. This would be a group of people consisting of physicians, local medical society representatives, lawyers, judges, business owners, workers (white and blue collar), insurance company representatives, local politicians, educators, low income people, etc. This well-rounded group would be delegated the job of arbitrating the borderline or questionable claims brought to lawyers. Their decision then dictates whether or not lawyers could proceed further with these claims. Perhaps many of these borderline cases would be justifiably determined not to have sufficient merit and the process would stop here (another cost saving measure). Currently, the plaintiff's lawyer and the defense's lawyer arbitrate the case between themselves to a point of mutual benefit. I say mutual benefit because both parties know from a cost-effective view what is best for them. This is then passed on or "recommended" to the other persons or companies involved. Since insurance companies want to contain costs and physicians don't want their reputation damaged, most of these claims get settled out of court. The consumers or plaintiffs, oblivious to the reality that goes on behind the scenes, trust their lawyer and are usually happy to get what they assume is the best settlement for them. What they also don't know is how this drives up everyone's medical insurance premiums (including their own). The current arbitration process is one-sided, unregulated, controlled only by lawyers, and continues to elevate the cost of healthcare.

For our third category of claims, good, confident, and ethically concerned lawyers would know that they have a legitimate case on behalf of their client and should have no fear of repercussions placed upon them. They should therefore proceed as usual. Physicians have to decipher many complaints from patients, evaluate their legitimacy, treat the patients appropriately, take responsibility, and be held accountable for their actions. Why not lawyers? Why do lawyers get a "free ride"?

Here is an opportunity for Government spending that may actually reap more benefits through cost control. Create these "Arbitration Councils" and subsidize the income of those involved. Put them on the Government payroll if needed. Make sure however that they understand that the more nebulous claims they let by, the higher their insurance premiums will go. Everyone needs an incentive or disincentive to "do the right thing".

Speaking of disincentives for consumers and lawyers, how about legislating a law that requires the consumer and their lawyer to pay for costs incurred by a lawsuit brought to court and deemed frivolous by the Judge? This way, the costs aren't shared throughout the system by those of us "doing the right thing".

The Need to Re-establish the Proper Value of Primary Care Medicine and its Doctors

Primary Care must be acknowledged as the most important component to our healthcare delivery system. This is where prevention, wellness, and good quality management of chronic disease is done. We currently are a nation that mostly promotes TREATING illness; not PREVENTING it. The only way this will change is if the culture of reimbursement by insurance companies to Primary Care Providers is dramatically reformed. Primary Care also must be restored back to highly trained, fully credentialed, and Board-Certified Physicians. If the correct incentives are put in place and reimbursement to Primary Care Physicians is significantly increased, then prevention, wellness, and efficient management of chronic disease will be done to the extent of driving down the overall cost of healthcare.

If we reform our current ways for the better as stated above, then Physicians also should be held accountable. However, hold them accountable for what they actually have control over. I have no problem with the concept of "pay for performance". I strongly have a problem as to how this is currently done and how it will likely continue to evolve. I have already outlined what I observed when I was working at our Veterans Hospital and how electronic medical records will be ultimately used incorrectly by the private sector insurance companies. What will eventually happen is that partial reimbursement for "pay for performance" will be withheld by insurance companies until the end of the year when they will determine (based on their "outcome measures") if the Primary Care Physicians deserve it. This will be based on whether or not the Physicians met or exceeded their pre-determined "outcome measures". The problem with this is that who will determine what these outcome measures are and how will it affect the delivery of healthcare? If the insurance companies choose the easy way out by utilizing and accessing the electronic medical record database to simply collect numbers and percentages, this will only paradoxically propagate the current culture of ignoring prevention and will continue to negatively affect patient care. For example, it will be easy for the insurance companies to devise a software program that accesses the electronic record database of all patients of a Primary Care Physician (age 50 or above) to determine what percentage of these patients had their colonoscopies done. Now pretend you are a Primary Care Physician that has repeatedly spent an extraordinary amount of time engaging, educating, and trying to get a patient to get his/her colonoscopy done but he or she continues to refuse (patients have a right to refuse despite your greatest efforts). What do you (pretending to be the physician) think you should be reimbursed for? Should it be whether or not the colonoscopy was done? Or should it be the fact that you ultimately spent hours in vain to engage, discuss, and educate the patient trying to get him or her to get it done? Common sense tells me that the Physician should get highly reimbursed for his/her repeated effort and time spent trying to convince the patient about the need for the colonoscopy. As long as this repeated effort is documented in the patient's progress notes, the Primary Care Physician has done his/

her job and should be reimbursed accordingly. This presents a problem to the insurance company because they would actually have to READ the notes to find the effort that was executed. This would take time. There is no software program to do this for them. So the insurance companies will resort to easily retrievable electronic data (numbers and percentages) to determine if the physician gets their withheld pay. The reaction to this by Primary Care Physicians will be the same (if not worse) that I observed at the Veterans Hospital. I say it could even get worse because at the VA we did not have the option to recommend to our patients that they seek care elsewhere. In the private sector however, this option exists as long as you give the patient one month's notice. If things progress the way I think they will (and have outlined in this document), the way for Primary Care Physicians to "play the game" (like everyone else) and to get their full reimbursement at the end of the year is to refuse or let go patients that are negatively affecting their "numbers". This is obviously not an ethical thing to do. Nevertheless, when every other sector of healthcare around you is lacking morals and common sense, why not do the same? After all, everyone has the right to manage their private business as they seem fit. Unfortunately, patients that have multiple chronic medical problems and patients who are not compliant with preventative testing will be bounced around from doctor to doctor and will suffer the most. These are the patients that need our time and help the most! Additionally, these are the patients costing the insurers and the healthcare system the most! Why is this so difficult to see? I don't understand how blind our system is! This is staring us in the face!

If private insurers adopt "pay for performance" models for reimbursement to Primary Care Physicians, I suggest that they use common sense. In the long run, they will ultimately pay more for illness if they don't recognize how to "measure" ways that actually promote incentives for Primary Care Physicians to practice prevention and high quality chronic disease management. When evaluating a physician for reimbursement of withheld money, I propose a random audit of enough patient records so that the truth can be found by reviewing the WHOLE record. Logical "outcome measures" should be used. Some of these could include the following. Were preventative medicine measures addressed and promoted by the physician? Are the patients happy with the quality of care they are receiving? Do the patients feel that their doctors are addressing their needs and trying to promote prevention and wellness (regardless of whether or not the patients are getting everything done)? Are chronic issues being addressed and attempts at improving the care for these issues being done during regular check-ups? How much time and effort is the physician truly making to promote well-being? Does the physician frequently make attempts at education of his/her patients? There are so many logical things to look for to determine the actual quality of care being attempted and practiced. A software program picking and choosing end result numbers from an electronic database WILL NOT reflect the TRUE care being given! Once again, I must reiterate, if we do not proceed along the common sense and logical path with the correct long-term goals in mind, we will get nowhere in reforming this country's healthcare industry for the better!

Summarizing above, with regards to Primary Care delivery, the two most important aspects to address are the ubiquitous practice of defensive medicine and the current illogical and diminutive way of reimbursing Primary Care Physicians.

ILLOGICAL AND IRRESPONSIBLE WAYS OF INSURANCE COMPANIES AND THE GENERAL PUBLIC

The general public needs financial incentives to promote their family's well-being. In all honesty, most people are greedy too and won't respond unless you give them cash to do so. In their defense though, there are multiple economic pressures they are dealing with and many are barely getting by. Why aren't medical insurance providers actively promoting programs to give people financial discounts for attempting to live a healthy lifestyle? Don't the insurance companies see that the healthier people are earlier in life, the likelihood of them being healthier later in life increases? This would save them money in the long run. Any financial discounts given up front will result in increased cost savings years later. If the insurance companies need to monitor whether or not consumers are living up to their part of the bargain; let it be so. Just do it in a reasonable and non-invasive fashion. I don't think consumers would have a problem with reasonable guidelines as long as they get to keep their discounts and pocket the money for their own savings.

Why does a smoker pay the same premium for medical insurance through their employer as a nonsmoker? This makes no sense! The policies of Life Insurance companies don't work this way. You get denied life insurance just for being overweight. You will certainly get denied or pay exorbitant premiums if you smoke. These companies do their own screening.

Smoking is by far the biggest risk factor in developing a multitude of chronic costly medical conditions. Some of these include emphysema, chronic bronchitis, heart disease, strokes, lung cancer, bladder cancer; just to name a few. I know smoking is an addiction. We must recognize this also and concurrently put into place aggressive support programs and financial incentives to get people to quit. Nicotine replacement products (like the nicotine gum or patch) have been made available over the counter. Still, why aren't insurance companies paying for these products if a physician's prescription is obtained? This is ridiculous and illogical. In this scenario, not only is the patient making an attempt to stop smoking, he or she is also indirectly making a statistical attempt to save the insurance company money in the future. From the insurance company's point of view, why wouldn't they invest in this obvious long-term financial gain? Are they that consumed with their own short-sightedness? Currently, some of them "act" as patient advocates by having some sort of smoking cessation program they promote. They, however, won't pay for the nicotine patch or gum! Where's the logic here?

If a person has a chronic painful or debilitating disorder and they have been through the whole gamut that Traditional Medicine has to offer, why not pay for Complimentary medical treatment alternatives? If I was in charge of an insurance company and this type of patient is getting more symptomatic relief from a $50.00 Acupuncture, Massage Therapy, or other Holistic treatment than he or she is getting from the $1000.00 medications chronically being taken, why not cover the complimentary procedure so that the patient can be weaned off of the pricey medications that aren't helping?

It truly baffles the mind the ignorance level that is so pervasive even within the relatively small bureaucracy of a private insurance provider. Who are the people running these companies? Are they that incompetent or inept? Or perhaps they are just thinking of their greedy selves. Also, why does Congress seem to have the innate incapability to recognize and address these issues? Is it perhaps because most of them come from the Law profession which we have already noted to be the primary cause of the healthcare mess we find ourselves in now? Remember, physicians, patients, and even the narrow-minded reactionary insurance companies are just the Pawns on the chess table. The lawyers are the almighty and powerful Queens that take down the rest of the players including the King himself.

On a society level, we must emphasize, expand, and take seriously the promotion of healthy eating and physical activity behaviors for our children. This should begin at the earliest stages in a child's development where it can be learned and embedded in their future growth. Childhood education begins at home. Therefore, parents need to take more responsibility in promoting wellness growth of their children. Physical Education in school needs to be taken seriously, just like Science class. This is where Government spending is needed and justified.

Too many of our children are traveling down the street on a motorized scooter instead of riding a bicycle. Childhood obesity is becoming an epidemic. Children are no longer actively going outside to play sports with other children. They are sitting on their couches playing with their video games all day long.

CONCLUSION

In conclusion, this country simply needs to do a few logical things to get our healthcare delivery system back on track. To unravel the mess, we need to first comprehend essentially how we got here. To put it another way, we must understand the evolutionary forces that created the problems we face today. We all need to face our greed. We need to understand that we are not isolated from each other; rather we are connected. What others do to ignore or promote their physical and mental well-being impacts the healthcare system overall and your wallet specifically. Therefore, you must open your eyes to the problem.

Since individuals have demonstrated over and over their inability to reign in their own greed, Government must step in to regulate Institutional greed without compromising our free market system. With a little bit of intelligence and foresight, this can be done. We have the power to elect leaders to do this the correct way and hold them accountable. Members of Congress are quite aware of the public's ability to vote them out of office if we need to.

Government spending is needed and justified when it creates programs that ultimately result in long-term gains (i.e. reduction of the deficit) ; whether it be through creation of additional revenue or improved cost-containment (or both). Individuals invest in stocks with the same purpose in mind (creation of capital gains).

The most important of all priorities is destroying the practice of "defensive medicine"! Without doing this, healthcare cost containment will NEVER be achieved and all other efforts made will be futile! The next priority of most notability is to re-establish the value, respect, and PROPER reimbursement of Primary Care Medicine. This must be given back to Board-Certified Physicians where it belongs! These two issues are rudimentary to the recovery of our healthcare crisis.

My hope is that anyone who reads this will realize that the answers are reachable and not that difficult to see when you are willing to understand and accept the reality of our own greed and how it propagated many in society to subvert and devastate our healthcare system. All we have to do as a society is to see through the smokescreen that has been created, recognize the few genuine root problems that exist, apply common sense, weed out the current elusive greedy players, enact efficient and fair oversight, take responsibility for our lives and our actions, strive for better health, and reset the standard by which we view others. When this is done, the system will fix itself! If our leaders in Congress are not smart enough to see this or are selfishly politically motivated and do not legislate with the above in mind; we need to vote them out of office as soon as we can.

I will finish by recapitulating my opening warning. If you want affordable quality healthcare and you believe that all productive citizens in this country deserve it as well, you must rise up and inspire reform based on the insight permeating this document.

ABOUT THE AUTHOR

Louis LoBalsamo M.D. is a Board-Certified Physician specializing in Internal Medicine. His career so far has spanned seventeen years. For fifteen of those seventeen years, he specialized in delivering Primary Care Medicine within the Private Sector and as an employee for the Federal Government delivering medical care to our Veterans.

His record is impeccable and his reputation locally is outstanding. Prior to Medical School and Residency, both of which he completed at the State University of New York at Buffalo School of Medicine Consortium, he graduated Yale University with a Bachelor of Science Degree in Physics. He has also excelled in the study of Mathematics and Logic since he was a child. During his Junior year in High School, he was ranked within the top seven students Nationally in Mathematics by the United States Mathematical Olympiad Association. He therefore has an unparalleled innate analytical and logical mind. Problem solving has always been his strength.

He was born in Brooklyn, N.Y. He grew up in the lower-middle class neighborhoods of Brooklyn and Long Island. It is this background that also provided him with much needed common sense. He worked hard to achieve his accomplishments. Nothing was handed to him. This uncanny combination of common street sense, an unmatched analytical mind, and intrinsic problem-solving capabilities, is what makes this author uniquely qualified to "spell out" and simplify the issues for his readers.

While in Medical School, he did medical research and published several Articles in Medical Journals.

Recently, he was listed as one of "America's Top Physicians" by the Consumers Research Council of America; 2009 (www.consumersresearchcncl. org).

He is currently an active member of the Erie County Medical Society as well as the Medical Society of the State of New York.

www.ingramcontent.com/pod-product-compliance
Lightning Source LLC
Chambersburg PA
CBHW020335290526
45785CB00005B/2024